"It's Not All Black And White"

A Survivor's View Of Life

by

Daniel and Marjorie Windheim

Bloomington, IN  Milton Keynes, UK

authorHOUSE®

AuthorHouse™
1663 Liberty Drive, Suite 200
Bloomington, IN 47403
www.authorhouse.com
Phone: 1-800-839-8640

AuthorHouse™ UK Ltd.
500 Avebury Boulevard
Central Milton Keynes, MK9 2BE
www.authorhouse.co.uk
Phone: 08001974150

This book is a work of non-fiction. Unless otherwise noted, the author and the publisher make no explicit guarantees as to the accuracy of the information contained in this book and in some cases, names of people and places have been altered to protect their privacy.

First published by AuthorHouse 3/7/2007

ISBN: 978-1-4259-7658-3 (sc)

Printed in the United States of America
Bloomington, Indiana

This book is printed on acid-free paper.

*I dedicate this book to the memory of
Aaron G. Windheim; my father.
Dad, your love and support will
always remain strong.*

ACKNOWLEDGEMENT

I would like to thank all my friends and family for their continued love and support, during the writing of this book.

Special thanks to Dan Mignone for his constructive criticisms regarding design and language; Jeff Kreis for his computer technology wisdoms, and Jill Nizen for her undying friendship.

And rose@roseillustrations.com for her great work and upkeep of my web site www.tbilife.com .

INTRODUCTION

The writing of the "Poem Book, Reflections of a Head Injury Survivor" was a bittersweet experience for Dan and myself. Expressing both our feelings regarding Dan's miraculous survival and re-birth. It also raised many other questions for both of us. As the years passed we both agreed that there were many gaps in both the treatment of the head injured and the services available to them. We jointly came to the conclusion that another book focused on these issues could be of benefit both to the survivors, their families and those providing services to them.

The following represents our joint and separate efforts as mother and son describe Dan's life and the events leading up to his injury as well as the ensuing years of growth and rehabilitation and Dan's life today. We hope our words will prove helpful to those who read them.

TABLE OF CONTENTS

ACKNOWLEDGEMENT vii

INTRODUCTION... ix

CHAPTER 1   NOTHING IS BLACK AND WHITE.......... 1

CHAPTER 2   THE EARLY YEARS 4

CHAPTER 3   THE ACCIDENT.. 10

CHAPTER 4   RECOVERY AND REHABILITATION 22

CHAPTER 5   THE STRUGGLE CONTINUES.................. 35

CHAPTER 6   GAPS IN SERVICE 46

CHAPTER 7   THE PRESENT... 51

CONCLUSION... 54

CHAPTER 1
NOTHING IS BLACK AND WHITE

DISGUISING WORTH

Words

In a gut; womb; soft cavities give comfort

The heartfelt, benign wisdoms
are like inner brilliance; shattering knowledge once again

jagged shards of wealth disguise worth
Saturated moments are top heavy, fitful, but not fruitful
In lemony rays, tinsels dangle; metallic are not charged
There is no worth in ideas, just
thoughts of cost, empty reasons

a life of ruse is plush; tender cheeks; shade
Without meaning or purpose, knowledge is not valued
empty phrases; utterances; stray aspirations
Giving us false meaning to existence, and God's brilliance
Gliding through life, we avoid His purpose and our tasks

Mom:" Nothing is black and white but black and white"! My son and I are walking along the Hudson River on an unusually warm late winter's day. As usual we are philosophizing and this thought occurs to me. I go on to say" of course there are zebras, skunks, and cats, but almost every thing else must be qualified. "A thought like when a cloud covers the sun and then is blown past revealing the hot yellow glow of King Sol. This black and white theory applies to Dan's life. Because of the fates, which created him as a head trauma survivor, he has had to move forwards to recognize the grays in life He has discovered, as did I before him, that gray can be beautiful- whether it is the river during high tide or the sky as a storm approaches. He was not always able to do this and this inability pre-dated his head injury at age 16.

To describe this evolution, I will share with you first the little boy I remember then the teen whose life was changed in a moment on July 3rd, 1979 and finally the man Dan has grown into.

Daniel will also write a section describing each period of his life

Our goal is together by describing Dan's experience as a Traumatic Brain Injury survivor and my experiences as his mother and number one cheer leader to create a piece of work that may be helpful to other survivors.

<u>Dan: Coming Together as one (or the Quarterback of my team)</u>

Now that I have finished my book called "The Poem Book" I see the need to create a second book. Not just any book but a book to help survivors of TBI (Traumatic Brain Injury) to realize that our lives can and do continue and will continue despite this major set back.

TBI takes many tolls on our lives and each residual effect differs for each of us. As each individual differs (blue eyes, blond hair) each brain injury's effect is different it may range from impaired physical activity, to a speech impairment to an involuntary tremor or it may not be visible to the naked eye at all and may manifest itself in impaired judgment. That is why TBI is often called "the hidden disability" An injured brain may not be apparent as say, a broken leg, but it's effects run much deeper

The idea that it's not all black and white is a concept that I have trouble recognizing at times. Since my brain injury in 1979 my view of the world has become very simple or concrete. I see many things as good or bad, black or white so to speak. At times I know that due to my brain injury I don't view the world accurately.

We live in a world where people in general don't always take the time to react and then make a decision. Add to this neurological damage and one's world is way off kilter. I do my best to live a good life, to dress well, act appropriately and treat everyone like I want to be treated. I live my life as best I can yet for me as for many of my fellow brain injury survivors, depression is common. Yet the consensus is that there are constantly new discoveries in neurological research and new methodologies are being discovered daily. They say that the capacity of the brain is unknown (supposedly we only use 10 % of it). From where I'm sitting the next 100 years will be filled with many new discoveries and surprises. Myself and other TBI survivors need to hang in there and keep working to be our best. We must persevere, and look forward to improved treatments and services.

CHAPTER 2
THE EARLY YEARS

Everything in Life

Everything in a blank space
My life, wide, lustrous moments filled to ceramic brims

While white is enamel, shiny in glistening mugs
This smooth, experience called life is
filled with stuff, everything in life
This, that, here, there, all, nothing ,black and white
Bad is good, good bad, all or nothing, sometimes all
Pain is sometimes spurned, sometimes not

To keep order, an impossibility, is forgotten, again

Moments in moments, are forgotten, in a moment
Like brick walls, they are hardly
together, hardly remembered
Hardy, solid, thick and dark; shiny
Lives consumed with everything, is everything and nothing

Mom;" It's a boy. You have a son". These are the beautiful words I hear through the anesthetic blanket I am under. As I gaze at my son, my first thoughts are, "You look just like Poppa Mark (the name my father has been known by since the birth of my daughter, Elizabeth almost 3 years earlier). He has a head full of straight black hair and a little round face. Of course, I think he's beautiful. Unfortunately his "big "sister, aged 2 years and 9 months does not share our enthusiasm. After greeting him appropriately with a kiss, she then proceeded to give him (or try to give him) a present of a small metal shovel. This was handed to him over his head. Fortunately no damage occurred but the next step was to put a lock on the door of Dan's room so no further presents would be forth coming, at least until Dan was old enough to defend himself. From the beginning, Dan was a contented baby who did everything that was expected of him, and on schedule. He sat up at 6 months, stood at 9 months and walked at 13 months. A happy baby with a pleasant disposition he fit well into the family constellation. Even his sister began to accept him. It was only when he was about four years old that he began to reveal himself with the strong character that was to mark his later life. This was mostly played out in 2 ways. One was when he would ask for a certain toy for Christmas or a birthday only to never have the gift live up to his expectations. The one exception was the gift of round puzzles received the Christmas he was four and one half which to this day Dan remembers as being his "Best", Gift ever. The second quality was that Dan always tried harder to succeed than he was capable- setting very high standards for himself even when these standards were unreasonable. This was exemplified in several aspects of Dan's life, starting as I remember as early as seven years of age. While every child wants to do their best, Dan's efforts always went above and beyond his skill levels. Needless to say this often led to his feeling frustrated. This insatiable appetite to succeed also played out in his school life. An example was when her was told by his math teacher in 8th grade that he should not be in the advanced placement class; he insisted he had to be. He was placed in the more difficult class and he did succeed. This was pressure placed on him by some internal master. In fact it never came from me. I was later to wonder at what cost did his succeeding in this difficult class place on him. This quality also came to play even earlier, as Dan was playing Little League Baseball and Midget football. He always tried his best and beyond. Often he would push himself beyond his skills and would be most frustrated if he did not do as well as he thought he could, or should, do. Of small build and stature with a shock of dark brown hair he would stand out in the outfield, intensely concentrating on the game so he would be ready if and when a ball was hit his way. If the ball did come his way he would run as hard as he could, his gloved hand outstretch to try and snag the ball. If he did he was happy and a smile would break out on his little face. If he missed the ball, his head would hang low, his eyes down cast and a feeling of dejectedness would take over his body. The same was true in football. He always went against the odds to outrun his opponents.

It was often to be noted how hard Dan was on himself. He never took the easy way out.

Dan was also the mischief-maker. He was the one of my three children who was always pushing the envelope. Like the time he and his best buddy Michael went sailing on the Hudson river in a small row boat (not a very safe thing to do) or riding on the handlebars of his sisters bike, down the steep hill that was in front of our home, or bringing home the scruffiest stray dog that no one else wanted. Dan was the one who gave me a black eye when he hid behind the bathroom door to escape my words of wrath when he had done something wrong; he pushed open the door as I was kneeling on the outside talking (yelling) to him and the door knob met my eye. His escapades frequently got him into trouble like the time he climbed to the highest branch of the tree in our back yard and then lost his balance, falling to the ground. Daniel was the child who had frequent visits to the emergency room and many x-rays of his little body. Fortunately he never sustained a serious injury until the accident that almost took his life and certainly changed him forever.

Over all these early years from his birth to age 13 were happy one particularly when Dan was about 8 years old and the elderly couple who lived next store sold their home to a family with 7, count them, 7 children, four boys and three girls. Three of the boys were aged 8,9 and 10 and thereby an instant boys club was born. Our respective houses became clubhouses, our adjacent backyards a recreational area and the street in front of our homes became a miniature athletic field where all variety of sports were played depending on the season. A happy situation for Dan.

Because they were such a large family, their parents were quite strict with the children and yet created a very warm environment. I believe Dan thoroughly enjoyed being with this family and often would feel his own family was somewhat lacking. Of course the grass is always greener in the other person's yard so Dan would ignore any of the draw backs of being in such a large family and instead, I believe, he often wished he was a member rather than just the friend next door.

These years passed happily for Dan as well as for his older sister Liz, and his little brother Andrew. Dan was the one of my children who would cut up at school to the sometimes dismay of his teachers. Yet he always tried exceptionally hard to excel in everything he did. He loved sports but sometimes would become overly upset if he did less then his best (or what he would perceive as his best). Still he would never quit and this quality would stand him in good stead when he had to face the challenges to come. At 13 he persevered and became bar mitzvah, no small accomplishment since he had to juggle his religious lessons with his sports schedule, something the Rabbi in charge took exception to. Yet he did manage to do both and on a warm June day, Dan stood tall in his new suit as he said the prayers that had been said by 13 year old Jewish boys for many centuries. Although he was later to question formal religion I think the values that the ancient scribes put forward were to become an important part of Dan's value system.

Dan: In order the write this book, I have to start at the beginning. I was born in Nyack, New York, a small town located on the Hudson River about 20 miles from New York City. Our house was a black and white Dutch Colonial with 3 bedrooms, a living room, a dining room a kitchen and only one bathroom (about one short if you ask me.)I lived with my parents, my older sister and my younger brother. My parents separated when I was about 8 years old. My parents were both quite supportive of me but there were times when I felt anger towards them for what I felt was a lack of attention and caring. My brother Andrew and I have always been close over the years despite the fact he is now living half way around the world in Hong Kong. My relationship with my sister Liz is complicated and when I later describe the accident that changed my life you the reader may understand why I on some level blamed her for what happened

Anyway we all grew up in Nyack, New York. My little brother Andrew was a B+ - A student and I was a B-C student very friendly and outgoing.

A great influence in my life was my relationship with my next-door neighbor, Mike Sommi. The Sommi family consisting of 4 sons, 3 daughters and 2 parents moved in next door Michael and I were 8 years old. We did everything together and became best friends. I valued the way the Sommi family lived their lives and tried to adapt many of their values as my own. I am aware that what ever I achieved in my life was the result of hard work.

Things never came easy to me. As an example was the goal I achieved when I became Bar Mitzvah'd at age 13.

I have a strong belief in God even though there are times when I feel organized religion is not such a good thing and serves to create differences among people. I attended the Sons of Israel Synagogue which was a modern reformed temple located not far from my home. Although I wasn't literally tied up and dragged to Hebrew School on Tuesdays, Thursdays, and Sunday school as well ,it was something I felt I had to do. We would march into the Carriage House each week, speak Hebrew and learn about the culture of the Jews, say this, wear that, eat this, don't eat that.

I often wondered if religion did more to separate people then to bring them together.

My early years were happy one filled with friends both boys and girls. There were big trees to climb, and nice sized hills to sleigh ride on in the winter or to ride bikes on the rest of the year. I suffered the usual number of accidents sustaining the usual bumps and bruises of childhood.

Before and during my adolescent years I found sports to be a great way to express myself. Little League baseball, Pop Warner football, soccer and Lacrosse in my first two years of high school as well as swimming, hockey and tennis as recreation filled my life. I also enjoyed watching all kinds of professional sports, an avocation that remains with me to this day.

CHAPTER 3
THE ACCIDENT

A sad moment

in my gut
raw and tender; gases, move liquid colors

Red turns blue, and blue moves
Down, down deep-------
To a place we do not speak
And it's never of

While sadness bowls, it strikes, hard and then deep
A blind sided, awareness, on barn walls
Beige, rounded ovals, are circular
Searing wood; cactus; stand like ferns

FOR THIS ETERNITY. WEIGHTED
SOULS REMAIN BELOW
Down, down in pain, consciousness sharp, sometimes dark
Blue like dark blue. The way blue moves, down deep below

Mom: The years passed happily for Dan with his only occasionally being hard on himself if he did not achieve what he felt he should.

Then came that fateful night of July 3rd, 1979 when Dan went out with his sister, her latest boy friend and a friend to see the fireworks in Piermont. I had gone to bed early and was awakened later that evening by a tearful phone call from my daughter. "Mom" she said," there's been a car accident and we are all at Nyack Hospital. We are ok," she was quick to reassure me. Dressing hastily I arrived at the hospital minutes later to find my daughter, her boy friend and Dan's friend were indeed ok. Such unfortunately was not the case for Dan. He lay on a stretcher in the Emergency Room, unresponsive to the hubbub going on around him. I was told that Dan had been sitting in the back seat when another car headed towards the boy friend's car and he lost control, went into a ditch and struck a telephone pole right next to Dan's head. No one else was severely injured and indeed Dan did not have a mark on him. However, later tests were to reveal he had sustained a brain stem injury, and now was unconscious and in a coma.

He was placed in the Intensive care unit where doctors and nurses came and went. Under the harsh lights of the windowless unit ,days blended into night and back to days. I was afraid to leave Dan's side feeling that if I did he would not survive. I took up residency in the hospital sleeping in a chair next to his bed and only leaving to take a shower when another family member or friend could stay with Dan. Each time I would leave him even for a short time caused me deep anxiety and I would rush back to his bedside, my heart pounding. He underwent a tracheotomy to assist his breathing but there was no change in his overall status ;the deep coma he was in failed to lighten. Medications were given to reduce the swelling in his brain. After a week, a consultant from Columbia University Hospital was called and the prognosis that was given was that Dan would survive but "would he be a walking, talking thinking man, there was no guarantee" Now the plan was to move him to the pediatric floor and this too caused much fear as I had become comforted by the intensive care nurses and the comprehensive care he was receiving. What kind of care would he receive on a regular floor? This was the unknown and quite frightening for me. As the stretcher holding Dan was placed in the elevator in preparation of this move, the music in the elevator began to play a familiar song, "Daniel" by Elton John. I was in tears before I realized it but then felt as if this was a sign that all would be ok. However, much time was to elapse before this omen was to come to fruition.

Days turned into weeks. Physical therapists came to move Dan's unresponsive body. Food was pumped into him intravenously and still Dan remained virtually the same. You could not tell anything was wrong with him for he had not a mark on him to reveal the brain stem that was not functioning. His temperature would rise to alarming levels and would only return to normal with the use of a cold mattress. Friends and family came and went; all would talk with him telling him about events occurring in the world such as the All Star Game to try and stimulate him. We brought a Sanyo stereo and played Jethro Tull, one of Dan's favorite groups. All to the same unconscious response. There seemed to be periods of time when Dan was asleep versus periods of irritability. Then one day a change occurred during these periods of wakefulness. Dan's eyes popped open. This however turned out to be even more frightening because this was not accompanied by any additional cognizance and the thought occurred," Is this as far as he's going to go?"

Weeks turn into months. The trach is removed at about 10 weeks into Dan's coma and he seems to be breathing on his own. Friends continue to visit and Dan's room is completely decorated with cards, balloons, stuffed animals and a large poster from one of Dan's friend's mothers who is also my friend. It says "When life gives you lemons, make lemonade". Who would have believed at that time this would become Dan's Mantra for the years ahead. Another significant poster stated "The journey of a thousand miles begins with but a single step. 'This too would be part of Dan's philosophy in the years that were to come.

12 weeks post trauma: Dan opens his eyes and this time proceeds to say to his grandmother and myself who were sitting beside his bed"Grandma, Bread" His voice is hoarse but the words are clear. Dan is coming out of his coma. This process proves to be a gradual one. Not like the movies where the coma victim immediately regains all his former abilities. Instead Dan needs to be reborn, going from a baby who cannot even sit up, to sitting, standing, walking and eventually talking. He is ravenously hungry and orders everything available on the menu. One day he orders 12 eggs prepared in different ways and he consumes them all. Despite his being fed intravenously during the coma Dan has lost a lot of weight. The Dan who existed before July 3rd is permanently gone replaced by this new Dan who has to struggle for each accomplishment. He receives increased therapy and the talk now is that he needs to go for a more comprehensive rehabilitation program. Different programs are discussed and my friend, Pam and I make many visits to various programs in the area. We are most impressed by the program at Rusk Institute on 34th Street in New York City. This program had been started by Dr. Howard Rusk in the days following World War II when returning injured soldiers needed rehabilitation. The feeling of the facility is one of hope and encouragement and so it is this is the program that is chosen for Dan.

Another transfer with its resultant anxiety is made, for Nyack Hospital has been our cocoon and safety net for the past 3 months.

We enter Rusk Institute and Dan becomes a rehab patient. As part of his injury, Dan is suffering from Dysinhibition, which causes him to act out verbally. He is placed in room with 3 older men. One of the men Dan decides to use as his personal whipping boy and is verbally aggressive to him. Sometimes he throws food at him as well and no amount of discussion is effective at this point to curb Dan's anger. He is lonely at Rusk for although I visit daily and other family come as frequently as possible, he is cut off from the support net work of friends that had proven to be so important while he was in Nyack Hospital. His therapy goes satisfactorily, however Dan is depressed. After 4 weeks at Rusk the staff recommends he be discharged home and that is what occurs. In retrospect I believe Dan required more in patient therapy and would have benefited from this. Now he is to return home and attend Helen Hayes, a local facility on an out patient basis. His therapy will include physical, occupational, speech and vocational rehab as well as a school program

Dan: At the time of my accident I was an active 16-year-old boy who was completely enjoying life. I was an average student and athlete, friendly and outgoing. I became friendly with a group of boys from my high school, and we spent the year hanging out, drinking beer (on the sly) and listening to Rock and Roll. It was the late 70's and the music of Led Zeppelin, Jethro Tull and the Cars filled our lives.

This new group of guys I was hanging out with were older and this made me feel more important. Mark, Paul, Dave, Mike, and Mott(who was my age) spent much time together going through the motions of being teenagers. Being young, and it being the late 70's , much of our focus was on girls, and doing what we could to have fun. Many Friday and Saturday nights we would get hold of six packs of beer or some form of alcohol and spend the night drinking and showing how cool we were. Many nights would end with many sick individuals, throwing up and/or making fools of ourselves.

On the day of the accident, my buddies and I spent the day as we usually did, talking about girls and enjoying the beginning of a summer without school. It was the start of the 4th of July holiday weekend and as day turned to night, plans were made. My sister Liz who had graduated from high school the previous year was working at a local McDonalds. She had a date with her manager; Charlie and she invited myself and one friend to join them at a pre-holiday fireworks exhibition. The evening is a blur after this and most of my information is gleaned by the stories of others. Afterwards I was sometimes to regret going out with my sister thinking if I had not, maybe the accident would not have happened.

Although I don't remember being in the coma, per se, waking up was not as definitive as you may imagine. In the movies and on TV they portray waking up from a coma like the individual had been sleeping or napping and now is awake. I imagine for some cases it might be as brief as that, but for me and many others, waking up was a long and heart wrenching process., For me being in a coma was a series of dreams. The one dream that sticks in my mind is that my sister and I were in a car accident and in the hospital (at least I think it was a dream not a memory). I remember being in a painful place where they make you walk and it hurts (physical therapy?). Another dream was about a little boy with blonde hair (My brother)? named Skip. He was talking to me while I was in the bathroom and people told me later I would often call out to my brother to come and join me. Waking up occurred over time so my memories are unclear. Another dream was about a beautiful; girl who asked me to be her boyfriend. Upon awakening she turned into a new friend who I had known slightly as the scorekeeper of our Lacrosse team She would visit me frequently at the hospital and I became very attached to her .

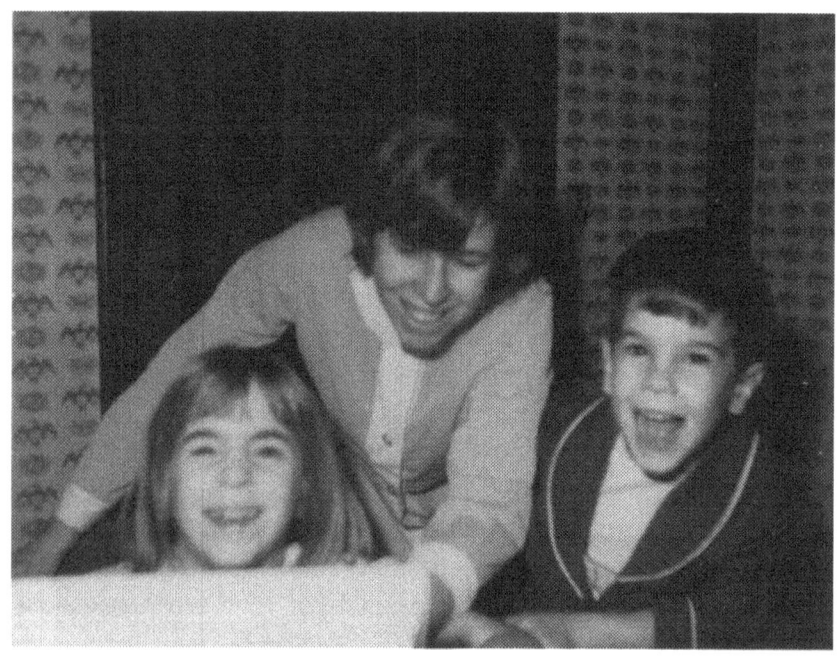

Liz, mom and Dan during 1960's.

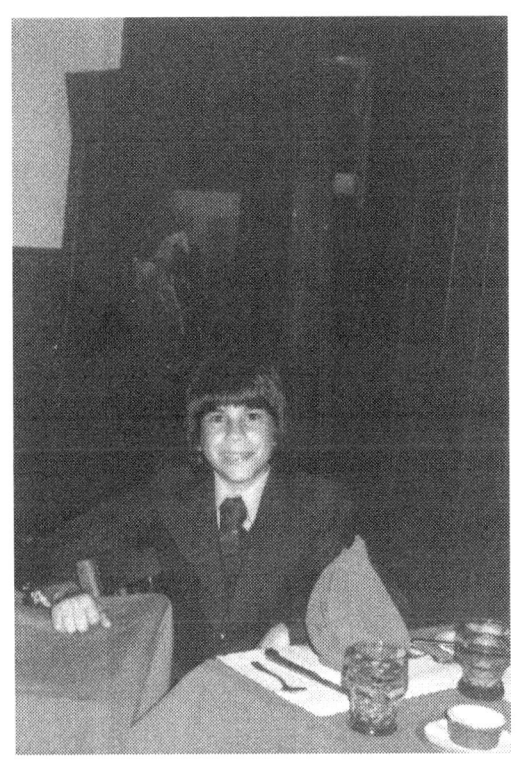

Dan at his Bar Mitzvah, 1976.

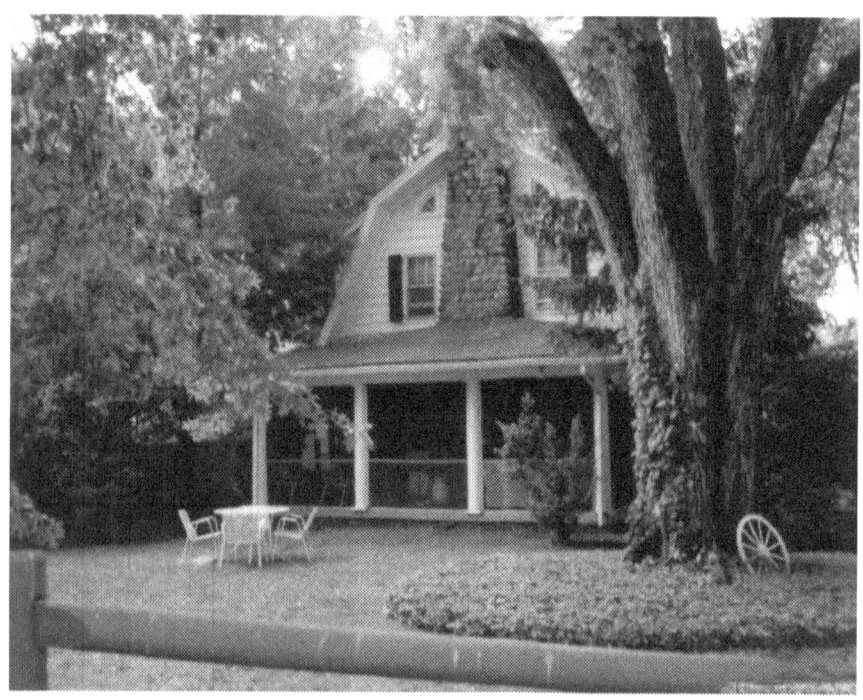

The Windheim homestead.

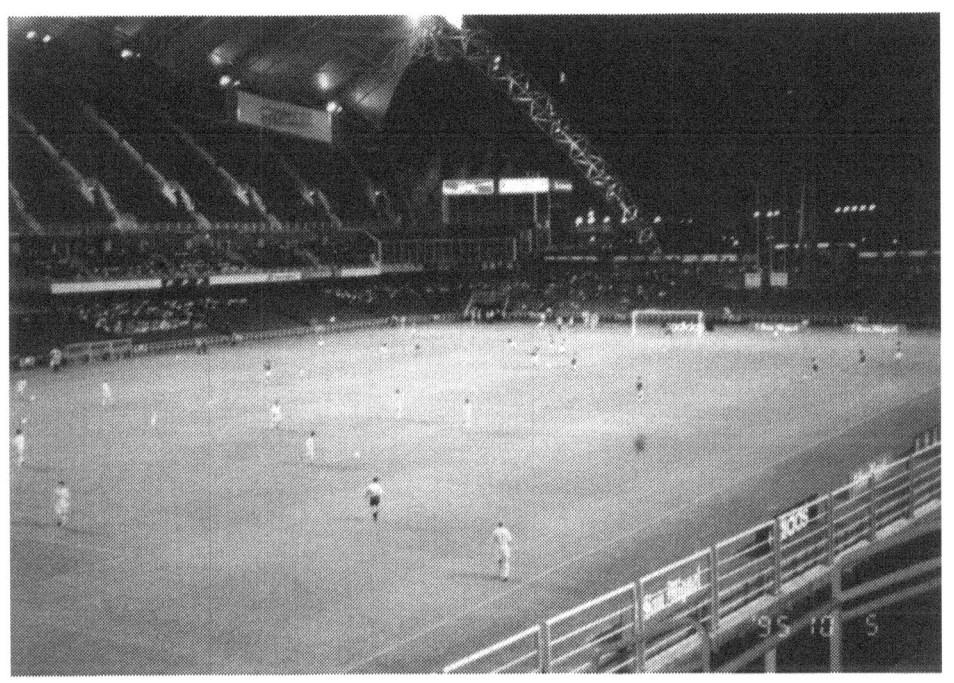

Soccer game in Hong Kong, 1995.

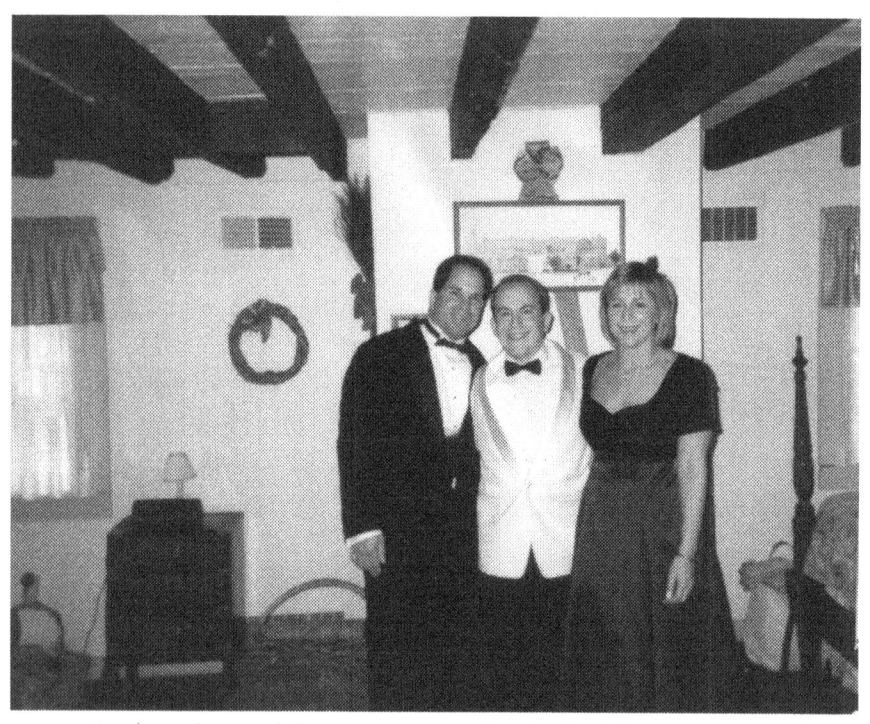

Andrew's wedding; Dan on the left, Liz on the right.

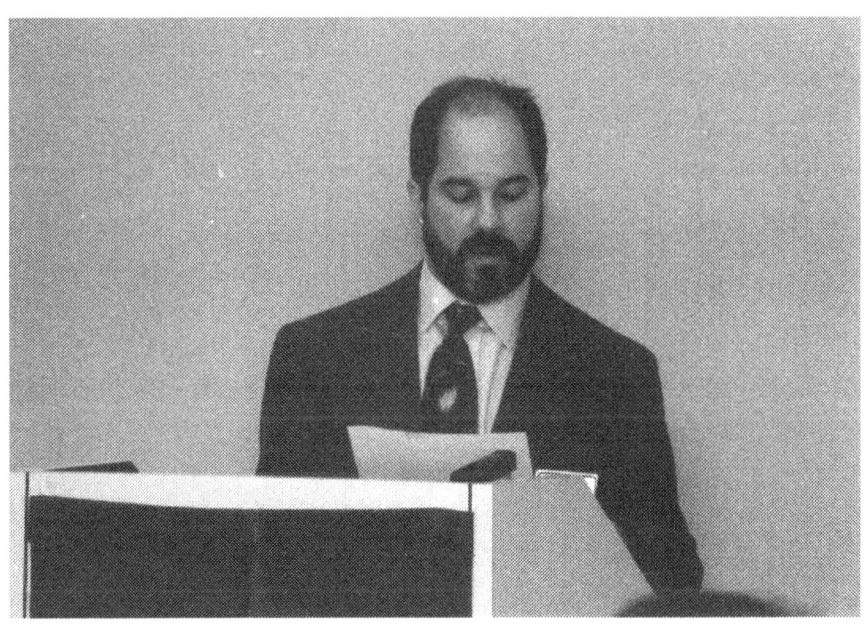

Making a speech in 2001.

CHAPTER 4
RECOVERY AND REHABILITATION

YOU GO UP

Slipping
loose dry grasps of touch
a sensory connection of gray fibers
smarts; of brains in life; like us

This lost bondage; truth, value, worth and reason
thin stringy wires to tangle webs of bundles
Without a known reason life is let go to get back

Like glutamate, clotting of dry cells
Running hard cotton
Narrow tracks, wood; dry of splinters
leading down to a gradual rise

for in life
You must go down before you go up
To success in life

Mom: Dan becomes an outpatient at Helen Hayes Hospital. As usual he works hard and by the spring of 1980 he is able to return to classes at Nyack High School and in June 1981, Dan graduates on schedule with his class. Many tears are shed on that wonderful evening as Dan somewhat haltingly but proudly flips his tassel to indicate he is really a high school graduate. These final years at Nyack High School are years that Dan began to realize the old Dan was no more and the new Dan would have many struggles. There was no more soccer or lacrosse and the overwhelming support of his friends that had been so prevalent in the weeks following the accident now has dwindled as they too note the loss of their friend and how he is now a different person. It is during this time that Dan begins to use writing as an outlet to express his inner turmoil and struggles.

What is next? Dan enrolls in St Thomas Aquinas College while he remains living at home. He enjoys following the college's basketball team and becomes somewhat an unofficial mascot. I become the chauffeur to attend some of the games as does his father. A highlight for Dan is when he is invited to go to Kansas City with the team for a Championship game. Living at home proves to be somewhat stultifying for Dan and he applies for and is accepted at Hofstra University where for the first time he experiences college campus life. He enjoys the experience but unfortunately despite the fact he is to be receiving additional support services due to his head trauma, he is unable to keep up with the work. Another college application finds him the following year at South Hampton College where he attends 1+1/2 year but still experiences the same let down as he is unable to successfully complete the curriculum. A transfer back to St. Thomas or STAC as it is popularly known finds Dan, living at home again, but able now to knuckle down and pass his courses. In May 1987, Dan is happy and we are all proud as he receives his Bachelor of Science degree. What a major accomplishment!

The next years in Dan's life are probably best described by him. My take on it was this was a time of continued healing and growth. Dan accepted a job as a counselor at an agency for the physically disabled called. "Barrier Free Living". This proves to be more then Dan is able to handle given his own demons to deal with related to his TBI. He takes and completes a Para Legal Course at our local Community College and is named continuing education's Student of the Year. He obtains his driver's license and attempts several part time jobs. All the while Dan has been involved with VESID and is continuing searching for ways to improve both his functioning and his quality of life. He learns and improves his computer skills. Recognizing that his TBI and the resultant emotional over lay gets in the way of his succeeding in finding and holding employment, Dan locates a rehabilitation out patient program presented by Rusk Institute at 24 th Street in Manhattan. This program is to change Dan's life for the better. The road to this change was not an easy one however. The program involved much soul searching, cognitive learning, self-questioning about who was the "new Dan" and how could he learn to cope better. As his mother I had to attend a monthly support group that was painful for me as well since I had to confront my lost dreams for Dan as well as learning acceptance of the "new Dan" whose expectations for life had to be changed. Many a time after these sessions I would find myself, walking rapidly by the Hudson River and silently cursing the counselor's who were giving me so much pain. When Dan completed two phases of the program, I had to admit that both he and I had learned a great deal and much of our denial had been broken down. Dan then went on to the employment evaluation portion of the program and this too brought new insights as well as disappointments that the post trauma Dan would never obtain the successes vocationally that he might have achieved had July 3,1979 not occurred.

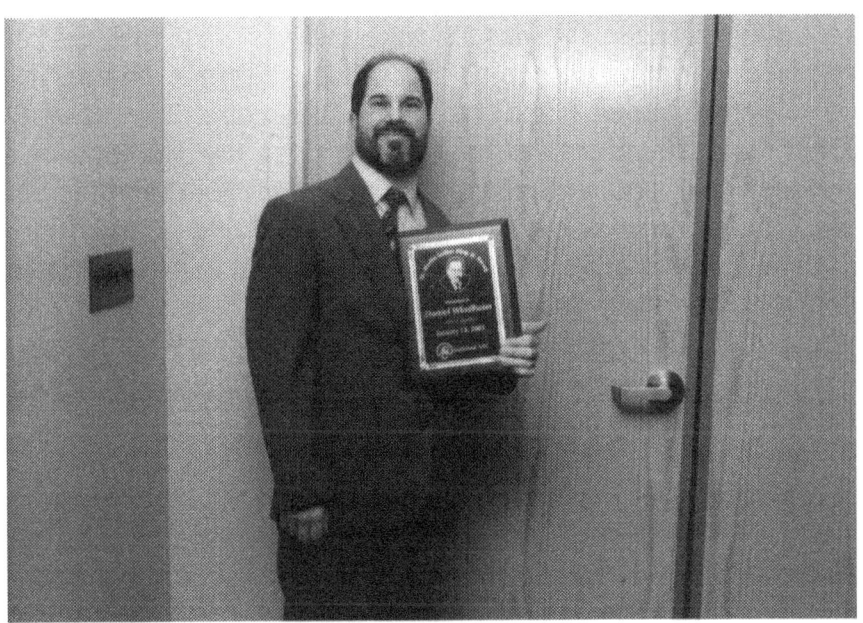

Receiving Dr. Martin Luther King Jr. Award
in January, 2001.

DAN: Living in Nyack, and recuperating from my injuries in Nyack Hospital, my family looked into rehabilitation at the Rusk Institute on 34th Street. Although, this was a long time ago, I do remember this time being a lonely and tough time. Being placed in an atmosphere with a bunch of strangers was both scarey and sad for me.

I was placed in a room in the adult section.(I was only 16) and had three men in my room. My time at Rusk was split between eating at my bed side and wheeling my chair (they kept me in a wheel chair for safety while I was re-learning to walk) to the elevators to take me upstairs to physical and occupational therapies. I do have distinct memories of some therapies I underwent. The therapist's were very friendly and understanding; listening to my feelings and suggestions , and making me feel heard and understood. In life I think everyone wants to feel heard and understood. I know I feel better about who I am when someone takes the time to listen and repeats back what I have just told them. Not just repeat, but really understand what I have said. ;this makes me part of my rehabilitation, and not just flesh and bone, a body.

My time at 34th St. was not all just work and rehab. I spent time going to watch a wheelchair basketball game, ; visiting friends who were patients or who came to visit me from outside; watching movies in the Rec. room (where I mostly slept); and attending beer parties in the cafeteria. Yong people in the late 70's and early 80's did a lot of foolish drinking before they grew up and learned the potential dangers that could come with it. There was not the strict enforcement of age as a requirement to consume alcohol as there is today I was to later learn that alcohol use is common among TBI survivors and yet is harmful to their functioning and should be avoided.

The Rusk Institute had originally been created to treat veterans returning from the 2nd world war.In search of better rehabilitation, I later was to return to 34th Street to attend a brain injury evaluation course to help me get a grip on where I was going in my life. Though physically I had recuperated quite a bit, I still possessed much anger and frustration over what I could not do and my mind was still littered with stray thoughts, ideas and unimportant information. This is similar to reading a book with a radio blaring in the background. My concentration kept going from the radio to the book and back to the radio. I was losing jobs, aggravating family and friends and hoping I could do better. After my weeks evaluation I was told that there was a program for head injury survivors on 24th street. I learned this program was a world renowned program started by Dr.. Yehuda Ben-yishay.

My life has been aided through a number of major milestones since my injury and each one has been instrumental in my recovery, but my work at the Rusk Head Injury Program was an invaluable experience. It was based on three major principles: Becoming aware of ones injury; compensation for this injury and acceptance of one's new self

The program was run as a therapeutic environment with participants sitting in a large circle around the perimeter of the room. All around the room were posters taped to the wall, with goals written on them for each trainee (we were known as trainees). Throughout each cycle each of us was to work on our individual weaknesses, and come to a point of awareness and acceptance through cognitive re-training,

Interspersed in the circle were trained therapists, neuro-pyschologists and other professionals. With their expertise and my "never give up attitude" I completed 2 ten week cycles (phase one) and one cycle of phase two, a work internship at NYU Medical Center. Although I did satisfactorily with the work, my relationship with my co-workers was poor, at least this is my perception, Even today I often feel my social skills are lacking I work really hard to be objective yet for some reason these thoughts in my mind fill me with self doubt. It is as if my self-confidence has been sapped away. Even when I know I'm right I dwell on my deficiencies. After a brain injury it is a constant effort to be on point.

Any way the work in this community forced me to compromise my views about myself. It seemed as if the neuropsychologists knew what I was thinking and based on this they knew what my actions would be; They knew just what to say to elicit responses (as if I was one of Skinner's rats in a box) They told us there was no magic pill to make us better and they would say things to make us react the way they wanted. Initially angry, over the weeks my anger was broken down and through coaching I learned coping mechanisms to deal with the new me.

One particular activity that was to try my patience and put me to the test was called The Hot Seat. This was an exercise whereby the participant of the day was put in front of the entire group with their counselor bedside them. The counselor would discuss with their participant about touchy issues that the participant was to be working on as part of their rehabilitation. This session often proved to be an emotional experience for the participant and was video taped so they could review the session later. The goal was to help the individual learn what defenses he or she was putting up to avoid acceptance and relearning effective coping mechanisms as a head injury survivor. The very name HOT Seat can give the reader an inkling of what it was like for the individual. To say this was a time of stress, sorrow, anger and almost any other emotion you can think of would be an understatement.

Other activities focused on eye/hand coordination, sequencing ideas, and working on tasks necessary for daily living.

At the end of the phase there was a graduation ceremony during which each participant had to give a speech. This was in front of the other participants, family and friends. It was indeed another tool of the program as individuals who had difficulty expressing themselves due to their brain trauma were called upon to do just that. This, although a difficult experience, was also a joyous occasion.

I would encourage TBI Survivors to seek out a program comparable to this Brain Injury Program at N.Y.U, a trip to the Internet searching out rehabilitation programs or a call to a local hospital or a state TBI group might lead a survivor to such a program. At the end of this book the reader will find a list of state agencies for their use.

What followed was a work evaluation that placed each individual in a work environment as well as testing them as to what this Post Traumatic Brain Injury survivor would be capable of in the real world. For me this was a continued time of learning for despite the fact that I had earned a Bachelor of Science Degree as well as a certificate as a Para Legal, I was advised I could not compete in a regular employment situation and instead was told to seek out volunteer work.

At the end of Phase 2 I was informed I was finished and to go home.

Although my new self was 150 times better off and 200 times more job ready (compared to the angry young man I had been two years before) I was still jobless and this troubled me. I often would express my frustration in writing and the following essays are examples of the value system I had developed for myself and the reality of what the head trauma had cost me.

The following are some essays, which express these feelings. Although I had been changed drastically due to my injuries; my old self still remains a great part of who I am.

Essay on Earl Campbell

I was born in 1963 and spent much of the 70's, before my accident, watching and playing sports. One football player I particularly enjoyed watching was Earl Campbell. He was a rugged, sparring running back for the Houston

Oilers. Earl came out of the University of Texas in 1977 and was the first pick in the NFL draft. He went on to win Rookie of the year honors, as well as being MVP. What I particularly liked about his style of play was that he did not shy away from anyone. Watch a football game today and you will see a running back run out of bounds to avoid being hit hard by opposing players. Earl never did this. He therefore got hit often in his efforts to pick up the most yards possible. As a result he sustained lasting injuries and his career ended early. I admired the way he played the game to his greatest capacity. He played each game as if it was his last. Asked today if he would have played the game differently to avoid such punishment as his body sustained and he says" No" He wanted to give every play his all. This is the way I try to live my life. I give everything I do, 100%. As I read in a book by Dan Millman, _The Way of the Peaceful Warrior_"" do everything on life the way Picasso painted, the way Mozart composed music, and the way Shakespeare wrote. Live each second like it is your last. I try to live my life as a peaceful warrior, with grace, pride and to be the best me I can.

Essay on Good Will Hunting

This feeling of guilt is overwhelming; it is all encompassing. "It's not your fault", this is what I try to convey to my friends as well as myself. This traumatic brain injury did not make us rotten, undeserving people. The words," It's not your fault" are spoken by Robin Williams portraying a psychologist in the movie, Good Will Hunting. As the counselor for Will, a troubled young delinquent, the therapist repeats it is not your fault, which ultimately causes the tough young Will to break into tears.

Back to real life. It is my opinion as well as the experience of some of my fellow TBI survivors that we are not deserving of goodness in our lives. Internally we know that we try to do the right thing to better ourselves and the world around us. But, at least for me, there is something that holds me back from enjoying life fully. I look at my life and feel there is something wrong with me. Because we may not look like, talk like, think like the general population, we are shell shocked into believing we are less then the average person. Like Will in Good Will Hunting, we are scared and need to let go of our burdens, and live life with pleasure in our hearts. Accepting this new self means letting go of the old self and admitting we are different. Although my pre injury life was filled with many valuable interactions and fulfilling experience, my new life also has its richness; I have a good mind despite the TBI.

Essay on exercise and sports

As a child exercise and sports played a big role in my life. This role has stayed strong and has given me a "never die" attitude towards life. I have always treated everything I do as a challenge and worked towards being the best I could be. In my youth I remember the sit-ups, push ups and squats that my elementary school gym teacher, Mr. Audervard would have us do. The goal was to develop our little muscles. I have always been under the impression that exercise is necessary for a healthier and better quality of life. At home my parents installed a basketball hoop in our driveway which became a major fixture in the family's life as well as for the neighborhood kids who would gather in our driveway to practice their shooting skills. One memorable trip to North Carolina and our only connection with the mainland was listening to the New York Knickerbockers on a small portable radio as they played an important game.

No matter where we were sports reigned. A vacation in Canada found us watching the New York Rangers play the Montreal, "Canadians." And also watching our beloved N.Y. Knicks take on the Baltimore Bullets. My Dad always made sure my brother, my sister and I attended various sporting events from watching the New York Mets play baseball, to tennis matches at Forest Hills and trips to New Haven to watch the football Giants play in the days before the Meadow Lands was built.

Over the years sports gave me a feeling of identity and belonging; I took pride in wearing my team jersey whether the sport was Little league baseball, Pop Warner football or later on Junior High and High School La Crosse and soccer. Even today holding onto the memories of those days makes me feel proud.

Today as a disabled person, much of my life is still filled with exercise. Now the exercise is important to help me deal with the results of my traumatic brain injury. The left side of my body was affected due to brain damage and there are gaps in the messages my brain sends to my left side. I tell my left hand to reach for an object and my arm stretches out but not to full extension. A good part of my work involves stretching the ligaments in my left arm (my wrist and my elbow) to combat stiffness and to gain as much of the use of my left arm as possible. Though you can tell there is something wrong with my arm I am very proud of what I can do with it. I do have a left arm and want to use it as much as possible. I hold a glass or cup in it, lift items, brush my teeth, shave and type with it. I also spend much time stretching the rest of my body, doing sit-ups and push-ups and walking in the great out doors. It is very important to me to feel good and look good.

Having a herniated disk has also forced me into doing a host of exercises, which were recommended to me by a physical therapist. I must do these exercises in the morning and at night if they are to be effective and believe me there are times they are a nuisance and I may have to force myself to complete this regimen. At these times I must tell myself to "suck it up" in order to force myself to do them. I know that the effort expended is worth it to make me feel better. I believe many people have trouble starting their exercise or even another kind of work but those who do reap the benefits in the end.

Throughout my life I have worked hard to meet my challenges; you can also meet yours through dedication and perseverance.

Essay on apologizing

I was in Barnes and Nobles Book Store the other day, purchasing a book on 'Head Injury, and I experienced something very strange. I thanked the sales clerk for getting me a book, and she said something that flooded my mind, She responded to my thank you with" no worries". What did that expression mean? Let me see, I guess it meant I should not worry about her helping me. That it was no problem for her to help me. Yeah, I GUESS THAT'S WHAT SHE MEANT. Then I thought about how many Head Injured People, including myself are constantly apologizing for our actions. Like we need to apologize for being disabled. DID WE DO SOMETHING WRONG TO CAUSE THE SITUATION WE ARE IN? As far back as I can remember since the accident I remember myself constantly saying" I'm sorry", for breaking an appointment, for a friend losing a job, for not calling a friend after I said I would. Now that I think about it, I am sorry, sorry I was in an accident and suffered a head injury! Not only for myself but also for my family and friends. I think how heart wrenching it must have been back then to see a son, grandson, brother, friend lying unconscious, clinging to life. Not knowing whether he will live or die, will he remain comatose? What kind of life will he have? A lot of grief. Still I don't believe a survivor should be sorry forever. Even if this is a human condition saying "I'm sorry" is very easy People have told me I don't need to apologize for my limitations. I know I am worthy and valued. Still I find I am constantly apologizing . In the book, "Don't Sweat The Small Stuff" the message makes much sense. Still there are many moments when I revert to my old patterns, get flooded and find myself playing the old" poor me" song and then apologizing yet again. I need to step back, think through the situation and remember **this** is a process and I must remember to continue moving forward doing the best I can. A survivor is someone who should be valued and who is worthy.

CHAPTER 5
THE STRUGGLE CONTINUES

<u>A SINGLE TREE IS KEPT</u>

Dark fluted skin casts shadows across rocks
secluded visions remain scarce but held for eternity

Babbling brooks that cause some to
return to youth, again and again
Others to draw or paint; visions are sealed into celluloid
Scars of life similar to rantings from
childhood, are wounds that heal

Like flesh gash caused by broken springs
of a soft mattress (is an irony)
Tiny yellow diamonds surround soft red and royal blue

chicken pox brings scratching, leave marks for life
Touched knees, foreheads, hands for that matter

The marks or seals that identify;
distinguish direction through life
Hard cartilage punctured to save a life, continue life
Blue, green, yellow but no red in a wooden shirt drawer

reminders of travels from that
mountain with a single tree

Mom: The year is 2001. Dan's writing of poetry has been a great catharsis for him. He now wants to share his outpouring of emotions as he struggles as a TBI survivor. The result is "The Poem Book: Reflections of a Head Injury Survivor." This project is to lead Dan into more endeavors as a public speaker and a marketer of his project. As in everything he does, Dan jumps into this running, enthusiasm and creativity reign. He also creates his Web Page and this open a whole new avenue of contact with other survivors. As the years progress Dan feels the desire to help others more and more. As he recognized gaps in resources for himself he also notices it for others. His question and answer feature of his web page follows and gives a clear portrait of the experiences others undergo as they struggle to live their lives to the fullest

Dan: Paid work is very important and necessary, yet over the last 25 years or so I have done much volunteer work of all types. "Work is work" and as long as you are able to make ends meet, it shouldn't reflect on one's value to society. I am fortunate that I found a part time job at a local library. I am also assisted by the government through some grants, the food stamp and Medicaid program. Because earlier I was able to be employed summers at a State Park I earned enough money and had a sufficient work history to receive Social Security Disability and after 2 years, to receive Medicare. I am very grateful that I live in a nation that assists people like myself. Giving back through community involvement is a small way that I express my gratitude.

Some of the projects I have been involved in were born out of my desire to have a place where I could be heard, respected and understood. Together with another disabled young man, The Motivators, a support group was born. We met at the Rockland Independent Living Center and the group would discuss personal philosophies, world events, troubling situations and strategies that keep our world together. As the leader of the group it was my responsibility to invite guest speakers and keep conversation flowing.

These speakers were from various groups of motivational speakers, representatives of local agencies, religious leaders and technical computer specialists who would share their knowledge and ideas with the group. We met once a month for two hours usually in the late afternoon. I found this experience to be most informative and rewarding.

Now, as I sit back in my computer chair and cross my legs, I affirm that at whatever age a Traumatic Brain Injury occurs, the effect is devastating. I have physical manifestations from my injury as well as cognitive damage. My left arm is atrophied and has a tremor, I walk with a limp and my speech is monotone from a paralyzed vocal cord. Brain injury does not make distinctions. Whether one is from Nyack, New York, or Siberia each survivor deals with their own problems in their own way. Many days I feel fortunate to be doing as well as I am and that I can deal with whatever life puts in my path. I do find that acceptance is a life long struggle.

It has been my theme to keep improving and overcome any obstacle. My wish is to beat TBI and live my life as if my accident had never occurred. However, I know now this is unrealistic and I maintain an attitude to do my best at whatever I can and the results will be acceptable.

As in life when one is confronted with a problem or "hits a brick wall" my responses or thinking at times gets altered. I might become "stuck in the muck". I sometimes then feel my life is a failure and I am a loser. I do not accept this new me. Yes I will live with this new me, but I will never accept this altered self.

Many years ago I began my own Web site, WWW. TBILIFE.COM dedicated to survivors of TBI. On it I have A Question and answer feedback form, links to important information regarding TBI, a section of poems by myself and other survivors and any other relevant information I can glean to share. I have found the web a key way to correspond with others and I have gotten feedback from web users all over the world. As a section of this book I felt sharing some of the responses from my survey would be informative for both the survivor's, their families and significant others as well as service providers.

(1) YOU KNOW THE WORD PERSISTENCE. WHAT KEEPS YOU GOING AFTER SUCH A DEVASTATING SETBACK:

Edna: To me persistence is the point of never giving up. I have not always been persistent but I am trying to keep on going, With God on my side, it has helped me go so far.

Kali: learning compensatory skills so I can continue to learn and grow. I have the rest of my life to master my skills

M: I use the love from my family and friends to keep fighting back to the life I used to live. My family would never abandon me. Several friends who are musically talented put together a benefit for me at a local bar.

Joan: I keep trying to set goals which keeps me going. After my wreck it was graduating from High school; now it is graduating from college I found no reason to actually give up. I think part of the reason is because giving up means death and I couldn't kill myself after walking away from my wreck.

Bill: I think what keeps me going is my wife, 19 year old son, my mother, father 2 brothers and sisters. I also live for my childhood memories that are so dear to me. I live them every day.

Teri: To attempt to reach my potential and enjoy a decent quality of life without regards to my disability.

2) AT WHAT AGE DID YOUR INJURY OCCUR? TALK ABOUT THE GOOD AND THE BAD OF HAVING IT AT THAT AGE.

Bill: I was 21 years old, in the prime of my life in 1979. I had a great job when all if a sudden my world fell from underneath without any warning. Well, there is no good in being injured at such a young age but if it had to happen, I wish I had been older so I could have enjoyed life more.

Kali: I was 38 now I am 46. The good part is that I knew what it felt like to be a functioning, responsible, competent adult. I used that as a benchmark for the functional level I wanted to achieve after I was injured. I think my recovery would have been more difficult if I had been under age 25 or so. I had to re-learn how to read, dress myself, work again, and take care of personal responsibilities etc. so knowing how adulthood used to "work" helped.

Rudy: I was 29. The doctor said had I been older the outcome might not have been as good. The bad thing for me is knowing what I could do before my injury and having to realize I couldn't do them anymore.

Sarah: I was 36. The good thing was that I had lived and had experiences to draw from. I also did not lose my core values. Physically I was in better shape than I had ever been in. I cannot think of anything negative about having it at that age.

3) ARE YOU OPEN ABOUT YOUR DISABILITY? HOW DO YOU HANDLE DISCLOSING YOUR DISABILITY WHEN INTERACTING WITH OTHERS?

Edna: Yes, I am open about my disability but it does get depressing. The more I talk about it the more I have to deal with it.

Rudy: I only disclose it to the people who need to know, or the ones I feel comfortable with. I feel that some people try to use their disability as a crutch. I went to rehab with some people like that and it used to make me angry to the point I would tell them to quit whining and start living. One person I keep in contact with thanks me for doing that for him. If it had come out of the mouth of a doctor or a therapist it might not have meant as much.

MK: Yes, I am open about it; I have to be because it was so severe. It seems everything centers around it; it is impossible to ignore I take it as just another part of my life. It does not disturb me at all.

Joan: I don't like to tell others bout my disability. I was raised with the attitude nobody cares about your problems so shut up and deal with them. I also feel like if I tell someone my problem they won't understand or believe me. I got a lot of attitude after my" wreck", about "you look healthy" why are you performing like you are, or that I was lying just to get attention. Because of that I don't tell people right away about my problems. If I get to know them better, I will tell them so they know what to expect of me.

4) HOW ARE YOU WITH ACCEPTANCE? I KNOW YOU ARE NOT HAPPY WITH YOUR HEAD INJURY BUT DO YOU LET IT INTERFERE WITH MOVING ON WITH YOUR LIFE?

Edna: Acceptance is hard. No I am not happy but I keep trying to achieve. Sometimes I take one step forward and two backwards but I have to keep trying.

Peter: I try to be honest with myself about what I can and cannot do, but I'm afraid I'll limit myself by thinking I can't do or accomplish something that I really could do; I have to re-evaluate my deficits continually. I have to admit I have allowed my TBI to slow my forward movement in life.

Joan: For a long time I didn't know what a head injury was. All I knew was that something was wrong but I didn't know what. Afterwards it was hard because I knew I was limited in what I could do but the fact didn't seem to sink in. I would push myself to the getting sick point because I just didn't want to accept that I couldn't do what I used to be able to do. I didn't want others to know I had limitations.

Sarah: I am very accepting by nature and always have been. Now however, acceptance is opening doors for me. I just wish others would accept their situations and get on with it. So many are hiding---- I'm not going to hide. I do not want the standards to be different for me just because I am disabled, but I am sure I will get them. I will find ways to work with them.

5) DO YOU NOTICE THE LITTLE STEPS YOU MAKE IN YOUR LIFE? HOW DO YOU GIVE YOURSELF CREDIT FOR THIS PROGRESS?

Edna: I really don't notice the little steps, but if I do, I'll do something like to treat myself to cappuccino or Chinese food.

Rudy: I notice all the steps now. When I started rehab, I couldn't do a thing for myself. I had a long way to go, so everything I did was a major accomplishment. I couldn't walk after the accident and then, one day, I walked 400 feet; that was a cause for celebration. Later in rehabilitation it's harder to see progress if you look for each days progress. But it you look each week or month you can see improvement.

Peter: Feedback from health professionals and friends helps a lot. I do, on occasion, re-read journal entries I've made during my years of rehab. It helps to see how far I've come. On the other hand, I see how far I have to go.

Sarah: Is there such a thing as little steps? Is there a way to give yourself credit for this progress without gloating and making others feel uncomfortable? My life is a series of major steps; I have overcome them all. TBI was obviously the largest step and the most difficult. But, I was not aware it was difficult. I just went with the flow.

6) DO YOU HAVE DIFFICULTY STARTING THINGS OR FINISHING THINGS YOU START? WHAT HELPS YOU WITH STARTING TASKS OR STICKING WITH THEM AFTER YOU HAVE STARTED?

Rudy: I have problems if I have to see something all the way through before I start something else. I have to write notes to myself to remind me where I am in a project.

Peter: I do have trouble starting things. I find nutrition and rest really help my mental focus. Vitamins, fruits and vegetables all really help with my mental abilities.

Joan: I have a lot of problems with procrastinating, I tend to start things and not finish them. I lose interest easily. It leads to many crochet projects half finished or barely started.

Mary Jean: Initiation is a very big problem. My attendant helps me by reminding me of the things I need to do.

7) WHEN YOU GET FRUSTRATED, WHAT IS IT USUALLY OVER AND HOW DO YOU HANDLE IT?

Sarah: If I start a task or I am presented with a problem and I cannot find a quick solution this causes me to get highly frustrated and emotional. I don't give myself a break.

MK: I get frustrated over the condition I am in. I just remind myself of how much worse it could be.

Mary Jean: I get frustrated the most because I can't work anymore. I try to keep myself busy by reading, exercising, watching cable talk shows, interacting with others and working on the computer.

Rudy: Myself. Mostly knowing what I could do before without any problems, which now I cannot even do at all.

8) DO YOU EVER FEEL LIKE YOU ARE AN OUTCAST? LIKE YOU ARE BEING TREATED DIFFERENTLY THAN OTHERS? WHAT DO YOU DO TO MAKE YOURSELF FEEL BETTER?

Edna: I feel like an outcast a lot. I have not dealt with it yet.

Kali: Some civilians take me less seriously and that is annoying. I have as much to offer (Perhaps more) as others. even though I may struggle with remembering a person's name or get lost in a new building when someone has given me directions to the rest room. I tend to ignore it, as it is one of the things I can't change. I chant the Serenity prayer a lot.

MK: I don't feel like an outcast, but I know I am treated differently than others. I know that someone who has had experiences such as mine must be treated differently. Not to expect that would be unrealistic.

Joan: I feel like an outcast all the time. I write a lot of my feelings down; I am not the kind of a person to talk about a problem. I don't have a lot of friends so I call my mother and we talk about what is going on. Afterwards, I feel better that I could get it out of my system.

9) DO YOU FEEL YOU HAVE A TOUGH TIME FITTING IN? WHAT SITUATIONS ARE THE TOUGHEST FOR YOU TO FIT IN?

Bill: I never have a tough time fitting in due to the fact that I could care less about what anyone thinks except my family and friends. If someone doesn't like me they can get out of my face.

Kali: No, not after all this time. I spent a lot of time in brain injury environments at first (support groups) but now spend about half my social time with civilians (church, community meetings.) I still feel best in a room full of people with TBI.

Rudy: Not really. The toughest thing is that my wife and I were really social people, going places and meeting people at events. Since the accident, I get tired quicker and have little tolerance for idiots.

Peter: Yes I do. Some of the toughest activities are with my 14-year-old son. He is very sensitive and I take great care not to embarrass him around his friends.

10) IN WHAT WAYS DOES YOUR INJURY AFFECT YOU? PHYSICALLY? COGNITIVELY?

Kali: I have a few physical effects. Balance is still not the way it used to be, and in general, I am less coordinated. My appetite has been affected; I have blurred vision, hearing impairment, and vertigo. I also limp from orthopedic injuries. Cognitively I have very impaired short-term memory loss, some word fitting problems and sequencing difficulties.

Rudy: Physically none. Cognitively many, speech, short-term memory, fine motor skills. Mentally this takes its toll.

Peter: Physically daily headaches, shoulder pain (broken in wreck) sleep disturbance, bad vision (almost lost an eye in the wreck). Cognitively much improved thanks to EEG (Neuro feedback) short-term memory difficulty, sensitivity to noise and light, and problem with organization.

CHAPTER 6
GAPS IN SERVICE

AN IMAGE OF GAPS

1. are lost in mind
2. The wide, barren openings
3. gaps, fig Newton thick
4. brown, syrupy and tightly packed seeds, clinging
5. Sweet is processed death in lifeless cellophane
6. Bringing to mind a loss of joys,
wisdom, lost to emptiness
7. The missing connection of ideas
8. Are chain linked fence-like, bonded wisdom once owned

9. Upon this huge mass, craters
exist where once bridges up
10. stood erect, polished with glistening brooks
11. now broken in silence, searching
tomorrow for vibrancy
12. tunnels and bridges, stretching thoughts to ideas

Mom: I will let Dan as a TBI Survivor present his view point on this important subject. Needless to say, as his mother I feel more could be done for Dan and other TBI survivors to maximize their functioning so they may have the most rewarding life possible. The unmet needs I perceive may not be the same as Dan's or other TBI survivors, which is why I encouraged him to use his web page as a sounding board.

From my perspective as Dan's mother, I feel more could have been done to give Dan the opportunity to use his many skills in paid employment. When Dan obtained his college degreee, he was given the opportunity through a friend's connection to work as a counselor at an organization that helps disabled people. Dan traveled each day into Manhattan and tried very hard to fulfill his responsibilities but after a month or two it became apparent he did not have the skills and personal self-control to carry out the job and therefore he was dismissed. In retrospect I believe that with a job counselor and more training he could have done a good job and been a real role model for others with disabilities. Certain agencies in our county do provide job coaches for people like Dan and it is my belief that these positions need to be expanded. Also more assessing of survivors skills and maximizing these in a paid position would be of help. A look at what contributions can this person make should be the focus rather then looking only at what are their deficits. Also survivors of TBI may become isolated and more recreational opportunities could improve the quality of their lives. Dan was fortunate to have hooked up with excellent services and this, along with his inner strengths and pre-trauma character have helped him to create a somewhat satisfying life for him. I do know that he has to work hard each and every day as he describes to" put him self out there" and I know he encounters both rejection and misinterpretation as he carries out his daily routines.

Dan and I have discussions about the need for TBI survivors to learn" acceptance" We have different definitions however. Mine is that survivors need to know what their limitations are and "learn to deal with them. They then need to look at what they can do well and maximize these qualities. Dan states he will never "accept" for him to "accept" means to say this is all there is and I can do no more. Dan always strives to "do more". His life is filled with this positive energy.

Dan: After sustaining a brain injury my life was turned upside down and I had become dependent on many people as well as systems and agencies to assist me in life. I was dependent from day one on others to help in many ways starting with doctors, nurses, hospital personnel. All were well meaning but at times their efforts fell short in my estimation. It is obviously impossible to meet every ones expectations particularly during the difficult times following a traumatic brain injury. It is said" You can't be everything to everyone" and I agree .One can only do their best. One of my goals in writing this book was to look at in what way could treatment of head injury survivors be improved To do this I once again turn to my web site to ask my fellow TBI survivors for their input on this subject.

1. (Courtesy of Anita) I think what is hard about recovery from a TBI is that there are few models available to help a person with developing a new life.

I have recently been trying to think about what helped me and what didn't during the 8 and $\frac{1}{2}$ long years since my accident.

I found a new environment in which it was ok to be my injured self in. I did this through communicating with and watching others with injuries. I got away from people who weren't supportive and developed a network that was. This meant working on my relationship with institutions. Early on the insurance companies were doing their numbers on me about the fact my problems were psychological (and they were real) I also centered my therapy on speech and language and found that rehabbing my deficits helped improve my emotions. I also felt a gap in services provided by therapists was affected because they didn't understand head injury. I was fortunate to have friends who helped me find therapists and doctors who were clear thinking about my injury

I have had to redefine my life goals because of my injury and now am working on "owning my disability" I was a PHD Economist before my injury. With my head injury I cannot do economics. I do want to help others with head injury. My gifts are my speaking abilities from my old life. I am using these abilities to teach others about brain injury. Even professionals listen to me. People tell me that I can say what they would like others to know. I am doing my life goals just in a different way than I planned or expected. I am not yet able to do competitive work but I continue to write and think about recovery. This is all ok and enough.

2 (courtesy of Rich) Maybe a program to form a job training program or other ways to make us feel more productive in life

3. (Courtesy of Josh) People are the key concern of TBI, Language can present barriers to our full recovery. Words can create negative connotations and associations that cause other people to see us as different or to treat us as different. If we can help others use People first language such as referring to the person with the disability or the person recovering from the TBI this would be a plus. . Also accessibility needs to be made real. Peer support is important and individuals should not adopt a victim mentality but instead self empower by using positive language. Recovery may take a life time but it is different then being a "victim of TBI" or remaining a "survivor"

4. (Courtesy of Rita) By finding resources within the community I can help other people. I keep a notebook with me at all times such has business card and phone numbers for most resources. These may be medical, financial transportation etc. The area of accommodation is a constant struggle that must be prioritized.

5 (Courtesy of Missy, mother of a TBI survivor) we love to hear my son sing and laugh. I don't notice his monotone voice any more but I just wish others would be more understanding. I don't enjoy being around rudeness and feel a gap is the need to increase understanding of TBI in the general public.

6. (Courtesy of Muriel) Many people are willing to learn and are open to meeting people who are disabled in one way or another. For many, however, there is a lack of knowledge and great discomfort at meeting someone who is different. I think the more that people with disabilities mingle with the rest of the population the more of the non-disabled will become accustomed to differences. There will always be a few clinkers who need to feel superior. I try not to worry about this too much. Life has a way of leveling the playing field eventually. Also the lack of a correct diagnosis by emergency room staff and your own internist is a problem. I was told I was ok and then struggled for months unable to perform as I did before until finally I received the correct diagnosis of a brain injury that explained everything.

CHAPTER 7
THE PRESENT

A future potential

White walls in life

We seek color
Livid personalities about
a fulfilling; an ethnic cleansing

We continue searching less hatred
Forensic prejudice is mistaken

We are not living with less fear
Gloomy days, with less love
Seeking love and beauty within our walls

weaknesses exist
The needless strength
growth hormones that grow

We just have future dreams, remaining
Silence of losses, mistakenly mistook

Leaving opportunity barely open
Possibility for end success

Mom: When I look at my son today, I recognize he is different from the man he would have become had he not sustained his TBI back in 1979. What I am aware of is how much he has been able to accomplish and as I watch him in the various aspects of his life today, I am continually amazed. To pin point some of his present activities, I would share with you his involvement in poetry, not only his ongoing creativity in dealing with the written word but his organizational skills in the work he does with a local poetry group that meets on a monthly basis. He has single handedly taken over the leadership of this group and monthly plans a poetry jam in which he does everything from arrange for guest poets, to publicize the event, to invite participants, every detail right down to providing the refreshments for the group; This is no small accomplishment for anyone, never mind a TBI Survivor.

Dan: All these years and no end in sight. I find this depressing on one hand and yet comforting on the other. "TBI is forever; there is no cure" I have been told time and time again there is no magic pill to make everything better, I understand that after my head injury, brain cells were destroyed and cannot be regenerated. Yet does this mean I can't live a satisfactory life. The past 25+ years have been difficult at times and not a trip to joyville.

I have spent these years researching and attending various programs, being a member of various support groups and traveling long distances to share my experiences with other survivors, I know now that TBI is different for each survivor.

For me my tremor is a big problem, mine sucks is the polite way of putting it. Life becomes very challenging and aggravating. My movements are herky jerky, nothing is smooth. I slowly move my hand to grasp something and my hand spasms and jerks forward. When I hand money to a cashier or try to receive my change, the money often falls to the floor. In the 1980s I took various medications for this problem but this did not consistently help my tremor nor did any of the other medications I tried. I believe I have now mostly made peace with my tremor. I have come to accept this tremor is not me but a manifestation of my brain injury. If I can put up with this nagging inconvenience I can deal with whatever life throws at me . I realize that because of it I have become a stronger person.

A thought occurs to me, how would it be if all people with a disability switched disabilities with someone else? I think many people would have more respect for others and feel less angry about their own situation. Like they say," the grass is always greener in the other person's yard.

CONCLUSION

<u>THIS WEB</u>

Is a tangle of words
Is like a list of non sense

I collect nouns, string prefixes, verbs to adjectives

Feeling shapes in sizes; colors, and textures

We create; I create
IMAGES OF PAINTINGS, THOUGHT
TO IDEA, FROM a VISION

A view of textures. Smells of depths; purity
WITHIN VISION, ALONE IS OBTUSE,
A PART OF EACH DAY

My idea of image is poetry; thoughts, ideas with feeling
They lift," heave-ho", catapult spirits toward heaven
Creating tiny spaces to unravel

I rejoice in life

Mom: What lies ahead for Dan? I can't say for sure. I only know that my son has grown from a boy to a man whose life was forever altered by a few moments in a car celebrating July 4th. The man he might have been is unknown but the man he did become is a treasure. He is competent, assertive when necessary, able to develop coping strategies to deal with the most difficult of times and yet is tireless when it comes to helping others.

We hope this book will be an inspiration to the other Dan's out there whom fate has dealt a difficult lot. I may have mentioned earlier the poster that hung on Dan's hospital room wall while he lay deep in a coma. It said, "When Life gives you lemons, make lemonade". Dan has not only made lemonade, he has created hundreds of soda fountains where both sweet and sour realities are dispensed and where along with the bitterness of reality at times, there are moments when people are valued as individuals and where there is always hope for a better day ahead. Dan wanted to create a follow up to the Poem Book to be of assistance to other's living life after a TBI. He and I believe that by telling his story, as well as noting his pre-trauma characteristics that have stood him in good stead over the years since his injury this might be of use to other survivors.

Dan never accepted his misfortune. He kept looking for other programs and support services, forever traveling new roads. He and I have recognized that these services may not be perfect but it was better to try and make these work instead of giving up and not trying at all. Giving up is not part of Dan's vocabulary.

Dan: I frequently hear." You are lucky, you could have died" People have difficulty speaking to me regarding my disability. I guess they are uncomfortable with me, recognize their own mortality, and realize how lives, even theirs, can change in an instant. But I WISH THEY WOULDN'T SAY I WAS LUCKY. I WAS UNLUCKY. The only reason I am doing as well as I am today was because of hard work, and inner strength to deal with hardships, disappointments and regrets life can be easy at times, difficult as well. It is my challenge not to get wrapped up in what others might be thinking about me. I work on concentrating on life, what I can control and what I can't. My word to other survivors is this, "just focus on what you are doing and leave the rest alone." Sometimes less is more" As it is said, "in the end your out mail box will still be left with things to do any way and that's ok.

If I were to summarize my advice to someone who has sustained a TBI, and is looking to ways to proceed in life, my list would look something like the following:

1) Find what you enjoy doing and have some success at, and keep doing it.
2) Try everything in life, even things you think you might not like. You might find you do like them
3) Be flexible. I know this may be the very thing you have trouble with but work to see things in a different way. There might be two ways.
4) Listen to your coaches, A coach is someone you can trust. They may tell you that you shouldn't carry all the plates in one trip, trust them and take their advice.
5) Show humility. We are all imperfect and do make mistakes from time to time. Learn to accept your imperfection and learn from it.
6) Challenge yourself. It is easy to accept the way things are. It's much harder to set a goal and strive towards it.
7) Be persistent. It is not stubbornness to try something more than once. Anything worth having is worth working for.
8) Don't be afraid to fail.

My life today is filled with constant struggle. I work towards improving at every juncture. I work hard to carry out my beliefs that nothing worth having comes easy. This has been my life long mantra. My effort and persistence make up for deficits. I never accept the status quo. Sometimes this can cause me frustration and I have to step back, recognize what I can and cannot do to make things better and move ahead.

Addendum:

Dan: I have spent the last 20 plus years working towards bringing awareness of brain injuries to the world at large, as well as making efforts geared towards bettering the lives of survivors. The Internet has been a key resource in my work. When I first became injured, assistance for the traumatic brain injury survivor, and even help for the disabled was limited. The present has seen a growth in awareness of the needs of others; the world has become more open.

To further that end, I am including a list of state agencies that may prove to be a starting point for survivors in need of services. This is not the end all but a place to begin your search

Best of luck,

Daniel Windheim

Since emails and web sites do change from time to time this list is subject to change. Do not give up; continue searching to find the help you need.

BRAIN INJURY ASSOCIATION OF ARIZONA
Phone: 602-508-8024
Toll free: 888-500-9165
Fx.:602-508-8285
E-mail: info@biaaz.org
URL: www.biaaz.org

BRAIN INJURY ASSOCIATION OF ARKANSAS
p.o.Box 26236
Little Rock Ar 72221
Phone: (501) 374-3585
Toll free: (800) 235-2443
Fax: (501)918-6595
Email: info@brainassociation.org
Web Site: /WWW.brainassociation.org

BRAIN INJURY ASSOCIATION OF COLORADO
4200 West Conejos
Suite 524
Denver, CO.80204
Phone: (303)355-9969
Toll free: (800) 955-2443
Fax(303)355-9968
Email: informationreferral@biacolorado.org
Web Site:http:www.biacolorado.org

BRAIN INJURY ASSOCIATION OF CONNECTICUT
333 East River Drive, Suite 106
East Hartford, CT,06108
Phone(860)721-8111
In State(800)278-8242
Fax:98600721-9008
E Maill: life@biact.org
Web Site http:www.biact.org

BRAIN INJURY ASSOCIATION OF DELAWARE
P.O Box 95
Middletown DE, 19709-0095
Phone:((302537-5770
Toll Free:((800)411-0505
Fax:(302)537-5770
Web Site: http:www.biausa.org/Delaware/bia.htm

BRAIN INJURY ASSOCIATION OF FLORIDA
Phone: (945)766-2400
In State: (800)992-3442
Fax:((945)786-2437
Email:info@biaf.org
Web Site:http:www.briaf.org

BRAIN INJURY ASSOCIATION OF HAWAII
Phone: (806)454-0699
Fax(806)454-1975
E Mail: biahi@verizon.net
Web Site: www.biausa.org/Hawaii

BRAIN INJURY ASSOCIATION OF IDAHO
Phone: (208) 342-0999
In State: (888) 3374-34447
E mail : INFO@BIaid.ORG
Web Site: www.biaid.org

BRAIN INJURY ASSOCIATION OF ILLINOIS
Phone(312) 726-5699
In State(800)-699-6443
Fx. 312-630-4011
E mail: info@biail.org
Website: www.biail.org

BRAIN INJURY ASSOCIATION OF INDIANA
Phone: 317-356-7722
Fx. 317-808-7770
 E mail: info@biai.org
Website www.biausa.org/indiana

BRAIN INJURY ASSOCIATION OF IOWA
Phone: 319-272-2312
In state: 800-475-4442
Fx. 319-272-2109
Email:biaa@cedarnet.org
Website: www.biausa.org/iowa

BRAIN INJURY ASSOCIATION OF KANSAS
Phone: (816)842-8607
In State(800)783-1356
Nationwide(800)783-3060
Fsx:(816)842-1531
eWebSite:www.biaks.org
email-liggett@biaks.org

BRAIN INJURY ASSOCIATION OF KENTUCKY
Phone(502)493-0609
InState: 1-800-592-1117,x223
Web Site: www.biak.us

BRAIN INJURY ASSOCIATION OF MAINE
207-861-9900
In State: 800-275-1233
EMAIL:info@biame.org
Web Site: http:www.biame.org

BRAIN INJURY ASSOCIATION OF MARYLAND
In State(800) 221-6443
EmAIL:INFO@BIAMD.ORG
Web Site:http:www.biamd.org

BRAIN INJURY ASSOCIATION OF
MASSACHUSSETTS
In Stater: (800) 242-0030
Email: biama@biama.org
Web Site: http:www.biama.org

BRAIN INJURY ASSOCIATION OF MICHIGAN
Phone(810)229-5880
InState"(800) 772-4323
Fax(810)229-8947
Email:INFO@BIAMI.ORG
Web Site: http:www/biami.org

BRAIN INJURY ASSOCIATION OF MINNESOTA
Phone: (612)378-2742
In State(800)669-6442
Fax:96120378-2789
E Mail:info@braininjurymn.org
Web Site:http/www.braininjurymn.org

BRAIN INJURY ASSOCIATION OF MISSISSIPPI
Phone(601)981-1021
In State(800)641-6442
Fax: (601)981-1039
E Mail: biaofms@aol.com
Web Site: http:/members.aol.com.biaofms/index.htm

BRAIN INJURY ASSOCIATION OF MISSOURI
Phone: (314)426-4024
INsTATE(800)377-6442
Fax:9314)426-3290
E Mail:info@biamo.org
Web Site: www.biamo.org

BRAIN INJURY ASSOCIATION OF MONTANA
Phone(406)541-6442
Fax:((406)541-4360
E Mail: biam@biamt.org
In State: (800) 241-6442
Web Site: http: www.biamt.org/

BRAIN INJURY ASSOCIATION OF NEW HAMPSHIRE
InState((800)773-8400
Phone: (603)225-8400
Fax((603)228-6749
E Mail: mail@bianh.org
Web Site: http:www.bianh.org

BRAIN INJURY ASSOCIATION OF NEW JERSEY
Phone(732)738-1002
In State:((800)669-4323
Fax(732) 738-1131
E Mail:info@banj.org
Web Site:http:www.bianj.org

BRAIN INJURY ASSOCIATION OF NEW MEXICO
Phone(505)292-7414
In State:(888)292-7415
Fax(505)271-8983
E Mail: Headwaynm@aol.com
Web Site:www.braininjurynm.org

BRAIN INJURY ASSOCIATION OF NEW YORK
Phone(518)459-7911
In State: (800) 228-8201
Fax:((518)482-5285
E Mail: info@bianys.org
Web Site: http:www.bianys.org

BRAIN INJURY ASSOCIATION OF NORTH CAROLINA
Phone: (919)83309634
In State: (800)377-1464
Fax: (919)833-5415
E Mail: bianc@biannc.net
Web Site: www.bianc.net

BRAIN INJURY ASSOCIATION OF OHIO
Phone: (614)481-7100
Fax; (714)481-7103
In State: 866-644-6242
E Mail: help@biaoh.org
Web Site:http:www.biaoh.org

BRAIN INJURY ASSOCIATION OF OKLAHOMA
Phone:(580) 233-4363
Fax (580)233-4546
E Mail: information@braininjuryoklahoma.org
Web Site: www.braininjuryoklahoma.org

BRAIN INJURY ASSOCIATION OF OREGON
Phone (503)413-7707
In State: (800) 544-5243
Fax (503)413-6849
E Mail: biaor@biaoregon.org
Web Site: http:www.biaoregon.org

BRAIN INJURY ASSOCIATION OF PENNSYLVANIA
Phone (717)657-3601
In State: (866)635-7097@
Email: info@biapa.org
Web Site: www.BIAPA.org

BRAIN INJURY ASSOCIATION OF RHODE ISLAND
Phone: (401) 461-6599
Fax: (401) 461-6561
In State: 1-888-824-8911
E Mail: braininjuryctr@biaofri.org
Web Site: www.biaofri.org

BRAIN INJURY ASSOCIATION OF SOUTH CAROLINA
Phone: (803)731-0588
Fax: (803) 731-0589
In State(800) 290-6461
E Mail: scbraininjury@bellsouth.net
Web Site: http:www.biausa.org/SC

BRAIN INJURY ASSOCIATION OF TENNESSEE
Phone: (615)248-2541
Fax(615)248-5879
Toll Free: 877-757-2428
E Mai: biaoftn@yahoo.com
Web Site: http:www.biaoftn.org

BRAIN INJURY ASSOCIATION OF TEXAS
Phone: (512) 326-1212
In State: (800) 392-0040
Fax(512) 326- 8088
E Mail: info@biatx.org
Web Site: http:www.biatx.org

BRAIN INJURY ASSOCIATION OF UTAH
Phone: (801) 484-2240
In State: (800) 281-8442
Fx:(801) 484-5932
E Mail: biau@sisna.com
Web Site: http:www.biau.org

BRAIN INJURY ASSOCIATION OF VERMONT
Toll Free: 1-877-856-1772
Voice/Fax: (802) 985-8440
E Mail: biavtinfo@adelphia.net
Website¨www.biavt.org

BRAIN INJURY ASSOIATION OF VIRGINIA
Phone: (804)355-5748
In state- (800) 334-8443
Fx-804-355- 8381
E mail- info@biav.net
Web Site: www.biav.net

BRAIN INJURY ASSOCIATION OF WASHINGTON
Phone: (206) 388-0900
In state- (800) 523-5438
Fx-206-388-0901
E mail: info@biawa.org
Web Site: www.biawa.org

BRAIN INJURY ASSOCIATION OF WEST VIRGINIA
Phone: (304) 766-4892
In State: (800) 356-6443
Fx. (304) 766-4940
E-mail biawv@aol.com
Website- www.biausa.org/WVirginia

BRAIN INJURY ASSOCIATION OF WISCONSIN
Phone: (262) 790-9660
In State: (800) 882-9282
Fx. 262-790-9670
E-mail: biaw@execpc.com
Website: www.biaw.org

BRAIN INJURY ASSOCIATION OF WYOMING
Phone: 307-473-1767
Nationwide: 800-643-6457
Fx. 307-237-5222
Email: biaw@tribcsp.com
Website: www.biausa.org/wyoming

Daniel Windheim is a native New Yorker, who attended Nyack High School, in the late seventies and eighties. In 1979, in the midst of his high school years, Dan was in a car accident and sustained a Brain Stem injury. But this did not deter him, Dan went on to graduate high school in 1981, and to later receive a Bachelor of Science degree in Psychology from St. Thomas Aquinas College in Sparkill, NY. Dan has been employed at The Nyack Library for about sixteen years, and is currently involved with his web site, which focuses on Brain Injury, (www.tbilife.com) He is constantly exercising his body and mind to better his life.

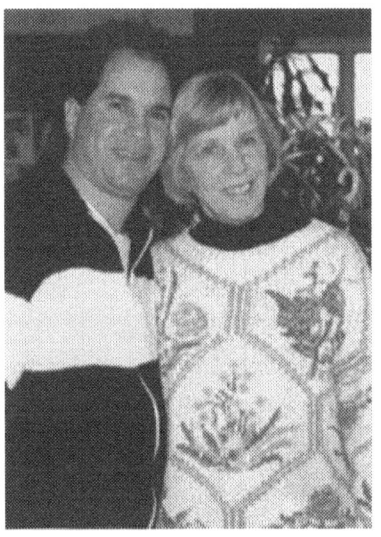

Marjorie Windheim was born and raised in Jersey City, New Jersey. She graduated from the University of Connecticut with a Bachelor of Arts degree and from Fordham University with a Master's in Social Work. For the past 28 years she has been employed as a Supervisor working with individuals, families and vulnerable adults. She has three children and three grandchildren of which she is very proud. As a poet and writer she was very happy to assist Daniel with this writing project.

www.ingramcontent.com/pod-product-compliance
Lightning Source LLC
Chambersburg PA
CBHW022132170526
45157CB00004B/1852